I0697275

GALLSTONE DIET

Creating a Meal Plan for a Healthy Gallbladder

GRACE BEN

Copyright © 2023 Grace Ben. All rights reserved. No part of this publication may be reproduced, distributed, or transmitted in any form or by any means, including photocopying, recording, or other electronic or mechanical methods, without the prior written permission of the author, except in the case of brief quotations embodied in critical reviews and certain other noncommercial uses permitted by copyright law. For permission requests, please contact the author at the address provided.

TABLE OF CONTENT

INTRODUCTION.. **5**

CHAPTER ONE:The importance of diet in preventing and managing gallstones................ **9**

    What to expect from this book........................12

CHAPTER TWO: What are Gallstones?............ **16**

    The types of Gallstones.................................. 19

    Risk factors for developing Gallstones............22

CHAPTER THREE: Symptoms of Gallstones... **26**

    When to see a doctor....................................29

    Complications of untreated Gallstones........... 33

CHAPTER FOUR:The Role of Diet in Gallstone Prevention and Management............................ **36**

    How diet affect Gallstones formation.............. 39

    Food to eat to prevent Gallstone....................44

    Foods to avoid to prevent Gallstones............. 47

CHAPTER FIVE: The Gallstone Diet: Meal Planning and Preparation.................................. **52**

    TIPS FOR MEAL PLANNING........................ 52

CHAPTER SIX:BREAKFAST RECIPE FOR GALLSTONES PATIENT....................................**59**

    Gallstone-friendly breakfast options................59

    Preparation instructions and cooking tips....... 62

    Snacks Recipe for Gallstone diet....................66

CHAPTER SEVEN: LUNCH RECIPE................. **71**

In conclusion, people with gallstones have a

INTRODUCTION.

Emma was alerted to a problem as soon as she awoke that morning. She had cramps in her stomach and a dull aching on her right side. She made an effort to ignore it and carry on with her daily activities, but the discomfort grew worse during the day. When she arrived home from work, she was exhausted and had trouble breathing.

Emma was identified to have gallstones following a trip to the emergency department and a battery of testing. Gallstones are tiny, hard deposits that develop in the gallbladder, a small organ situated behind the liver, the doctor explained. Gallstones can develop when the bile produced by the gallbladder contains too much cholesterol or other chemicals. Bile is a fluid that aids in the digestion of fat.

Emma was happy to get a diagnosis at last, but she was also anxious. From friends and family members who had endured grueling surgery to remove their gallbladders, she had heard horror stories. She didn't want to experience it, but she also had no idea how to stop it.

Emma then learned about the gallstone diet. She discovered that by adopting a few easy dietary adjustments, she may perhaps skip surgery completely and lower her chance of acquiring new gallstones. She jumped right into learning which foods were best to eat and which ones to stay away from, and she soon came up with a meal plan that worked for her.

Emma observed a tremendous improvement in her symptoms as she adhered to the diet. She was able to continue her regular activities once the discomfort lessened. She came to the realization that she had taken her health for granted and that even modest adjustments to her food and way of life might have a big effect on how she felt.

Emma's experience motivated her to impart her knowledge to anyone who might be dealing with gallstones. She offers a thorough explanation of the gallstone diet in this book, outlining the best foods to consume, those to avoid, and lifestyle adjustments that can support gallbladder health. This book is a priceless tool that may assist you in taking charge of your health, whether you have gallstones yourself or you just want to enhance your general health.

CHAPTER ONE: The importance of diet in preventing and managing gallstones.

Too much cholesterol or other compounds may be present in the bile of the gallbladder, which can cause crystallization and the formation of hard deposits. A balanced diet can lower the chance of developing gallstones by preventing the buildup of these chemicals.

Gallstones can be avoided with a diet that is high in fiber and low in fat. This is due to the possibility of gallstone formation as a result of cholesterol absorption into the circulation, which can be prevented by fiber's ability to bind to cholesterol in the digestive system. A low-fat diet can also lessen the liver's ability to produce cholesterol, which can assist to avoid the development of gallstones.

Dietary adjustments can assist those who already have gallstones manage their symptoms and avoid complications. A low-fat diet can encourage weight reduction and lower the risk of consequences from obesity while also lowering the likelihood of painful gallbladder attacks.

Water intake, alcohol consumption, and vitamin and mineral intake are other dietary variables that might affect the development and treatment of gallstones. While excessive alcohol intake might raise the chance of getting gallstones, maintaining good hydration can assist to avoid the formation of gallstones. Gallstone development risk can be decreased by getting enough vitamins and minerals, such as calcium and vitamin D.

Gallstones may be prevented from forming and their symptoms can be controlled in people who already have them by eating a nutritious diet that is high in fiber, low in fat, and rich in vitamins and minerals. People can lower their chance of having gallstones and improve their general health and wellbeing by changing their diet and leading a healthy lifestyle.

What to expect from this book.

If you are reading "Gallstone Diet," you are probably interested in making dietary adjustments to prevent or treat gallstones. This book intends to provide you thorough knowledge about gallstones, including information on their causes, symptoms, diagnosis, and available treatments. The book focuses in particular on how food might help prevent and treat gallstones.

The book is divided into seven chapters, each of which discusses a distinct topic related to managing food and gallstones. An overview of gallstones, including their etiology, symptoms, and risk factors, is given in the first few chapters. You may utilize this knowledge to create an efficient eating plan by having a better understanding of gallstones and how they occur.

The book then examines how food might help prevent and treat gallstones in later chapters. This includes advice on meal planning, proper cooking methods, and how to read nutrition labels. It also contains information on the kinds of foods that might encourage or prevent the production of gallstones. A large variety of recipes in the book are also created expressly to be gallstone-friendly, making it simple to incorporate good eating practices into your everyday routine.

The book also discusses additional lifestyle modifications that can aid in the prevention and management of gallstones in addition to dietary considerations. This includes advice on how to handle stress, deal with it physically, and stop smoking and drinking too much alcohol.

Evidence-based guidelines and straightforward guidance that may be readily implemented into your everyday routine are strongly emphasized throughout the book. Readers of various levels of expertise and knowledge may access the book since it is presented in simple, understandable language.

You may anticipate having a thorough grasp of gallstones and how diet can help prevent and manage them by the time the book is finished. You will have access to a wealth of knowledge that will enable you to make wise decisions about your food and way of life, including helpful advice and recipes. This book is a helpful tool that may assist you in reaching your objectives, whether you're trying to avoid gallstones or manage the symptoms of an underlying illness.

CHAPTER TWO: What are Gallstones?.

The gallbladder, a little pear-shaped organ situated in the upper right belly directly under the liver, is where gallstones, which are tiny, hard deposits, develop. By storing and releasing bile, a substance that aids in the breakdown of lipids in the small intestine, the gallbladder plays a significant part in digestion.

When the bile in the gallbladder contains too much cholesterol or other chemicals, the crystals can develop and harden into gallstones. These deposits might be little grains or massive stones with a diameter of several centimeters.

Gallstones can be divided into two categories: pigment stones and cholesterol stones. The most typical sort of stones are cholesterol ones, which develop when the gallbladder's bile contains too much cholesterol. Pigment stones, which are less frequent, develop when the bile includes an excessive amount of bilirubin, a byproduct of the body's breakdown of red blood cells.

Being a woman, being older than 40, being overweight or obese, having a family history of gallstones, and having certain medical problems like diabetes or liver disease are all risk factors for getting gallstones. The risk of gallstone development can also be increased by several drugs, such as estrogen treatment.

Gallstone symptoms might vary, but most frequently include upper right abdominal discomfort, nausea, vomiting, fever, and jaundice (a yellowing of the skin and eyes). Gallstones may occasionally go completely unnoticed and only become apparent during imaging tests ordered for another reason.

The intensity of the symptoms, the size, and the placement of the stones all influence how to treat gallstones. Medication and dietary modifications might occasionally assist in managing symptoms and avoiding problems. Surgery could be required in other circumstances to remove the gallbladder or the stones itself.

That's gallstones are minute, hard deposits that develop in the gallbladder and can result in a variety of signs and symptoms. Being a woman, being older than 40, being overweight or obese, and having specific medical problems are all risk factors for getting gallstones. Depending on the severity of the symptoms, gallstones may require surgery, medication, or dietary adjustments.

The types of Gallstones.

Gallstones can be divided into two categories: pigment stones and cholesterol stones.

Gallstones of any kind are quite prevalent, with cholesterol stones making up around 80% of all instances. These stones often have a yellow or green appearance and are composed of hardened cholesterol. When the gallbladder's bile has too much cholesterol, it can crystallize and become solid deposits, which results in cholesterol stones. Being a woman, being overweight or obese, eating a diet rich in fat and low in fiber, and having a family history of gallstones are all risk factors for developing cholesterol stones.

On the other hand, pigment stones, which make up around 20% of gallstones, are less frequent. Bilirubin, a waste product created as the body breaks down red blood cells, makes up these stones. Pigment stones are more frequently discovered in persons with specific medical disorders, such as cirrhosis, sickle cell anemia, and biliary tract infections. They typically have a black or brown appearance. Those who have had bariatric surgery, which modifies the natural flow of bile, are also susceptible to developing them.

There are more uncommon varieties of gallstones in addition to these two common ones, including mixed stones, which include pigment and cholesterol stones, and calcified gallstones, which are hardened stones that have developed calcification over time. These kinds of stones are rarer and typically need more specialist care.

Gallstones can range in size from small grains to enormous stones that might be several centimeters in diameter, which is an essential fact to keep in mind. The intensity of symptoms and the kind of therapy needed can both be influenced by the size and placement of the stones. Gallstones may occasionally go completely unnoticed and only become apparent during imaging tests ordered for another reason.

Risk factors for developing Gallstones

Millions of individuals all around the world suffer from the common medical disease known as gallstones. There are a number of risk factors that have been discovered, despite the fact that the precise etiology of gallstones is not entirely known. Individuals can take action to prevent gallstones from forming or to manage the problem if it occurs if they are aware of these risk factors.

Age is one of the major risk factors for gallstone development. Those over the age of 40 are more likely to develop gallstones, and the risk rises with age. This could be brought on by changes in hormone levels and metabolism that come with aging.

Another important risk factor for gallstones is gender. Gallstones are more common in women than in males, and the risk rises with age. This could be because estrogen, a hormone that is more common in women, can raise the level of cholesterol in the bile, which can result in gallstone development.

Another significant risk factor for gallstones is obesity. Gallstones are more likely to form in overweight or obese people than in people who are at a healthy weight. This may be so because having too much body fat can raise the quantity of cholesterol in the bile, which can cause gallstones to develop.

A significant contributor to the formation of gallstones is diet. A diet with a lot of fat and little fiber might make you more likely to have gallstones. This is due to the fact that a diet heavy in fat can raise the bile's cholesterol content, whilst a diet poor in fiber can obstruct the bile's natural flow and increase the risk of gallstone development.

A family history of the ailment, certain medical disorders including diabetes, liver disease, and inflammatory bowel disease, as well as specific medicines like estrogen treatment and cholesterol-lowering medications, are additional risk factors for gallstones.

CHAPTER THREE: Symptoms of Gallstones

Gallstones are a common medical condition that can cause a range of symptoms. Some people with gallstones may not experience any symptoms, while others may experience severe pain and discomfort. Understanding the symptoms of gallstones can help individuals recognize the condition and seek appropriate treatment.

One of the most common symptoms of gallstones is pain in the upper right side of the abdomen. This pain may be severe and can come on suddenly or gradually. The pain may also radiate to the back, chest, or shoulder. The pain may be triggered by eating a meal, especially a high-fat meal, and may last for several hours.

Other common symptoms of gallstones include nausea and vomiting. These symptoms may be triggered by the pain associated with gallstones, or they may be caused by the blockage of the bile duct, which can interfere with the normal digestion process.

Jaundice, a yellowing of the skin and eyes, can also be a symptom of gallstones. This occurs when the bile duct becomes blocked by a gallstone, which can cause a buildup of bilirubin in the body.

In some cases, gallstones may cause a fever and chills. This may be a sign of an infection in the gallbladder or bile duct, which can occur when a gallstone blocks the normal flow of bile.

Less common symptoms of gallstones may include a feeling of fullness or bloating, indigestion, and diarrhea. These symptoms may be caused by the disruption of the normal digestion process.

It is important to note that not everyone with gallstones will experience symptoms. In fact, many people may have gallstones without even knowing it. These "silent" gallstones are often discovered during imaging tests performed for other reasons.

If you experience any symptoms of gallstones, it is important to seek medical attention. In some cases, gallstones can lead to serious complications, such as inflammation of the gallbladder or pancreas, or a blockage of the bile duct. Early detection and treatment can help to prevent these complications and improve outcomes.

When to see a doctor

The symptoms of gallstones, a common illness that can result in anything from little discomfort to severe pain and problems, might vary. Knowing when to visit a doctor for an assessment and treatment if you are exhibiting gallstone symptoms is crucial.

Pain in the upper right side of the abdomen is one of the most typical signs of gallstones. The onset of this pain might be abrupt or gradual, and it may be severe. The back, chest, or shoulder might also get affected by the ache. Eating a meal, especially one heavy in fat, may cause the discomfort, which might linger for many hours.

Gallstones can frequently cause nausea and vomiting as symptoms. The discomfort brought on by gallstones may cause these symptoms to appear, or a bile duct obstruction, which can obstruct regular digestion, may be to blame.

Gallstones can also show symptoms like jaundice, which is a yellowing of the skin and eyes. This happens when a gallstone blocks the bile duct, which can result in an accumulation of bilirubin in the body.

Gallstones can occasionally result in fever and chills. This might indicate an infection in the bile duct or gallbladder, which can happen when a gallstone obstructs the regular flow of bile.

Gallstones can also cause less frequent symptoms including bloating, gas, and diarrhea. The interruption of the regular digestive process may be the source of these symptoms.

It is crucial to consult a doctor for an assessment and treatment if you are suffering any of these symptoms. Gallstones can occasionally result in significant side effects such pancreatitis, gallbladder inflammation, and bile duct obstruction. These problems can be avoided and results can be improved with early diagnosis and treatment.

If you suffer severe or prolonged pain or if you have any other symptoms that are worrying you, it is very crucial to get medical help immediately soon. This might be a symptom of a more serious ailment that needs immediate medical care.

The medical professional may do a physical examination, inquire about your symptoms, and suggest testing like an ultrasound or blood tests to identify gallstones during a visit. Gallstones can be treated by altering food and lifestyle, using drugs to dissolve the stones, or, in certain circumstances, having the gallbladder surgically removed.

It's critical to adhere to your doctor's treatment recommendations and show up for follow-up appointments so that your health can be monitored. The majority of persons with gallstones may achieve positive results and prevent problems with the right care and management.

Complications of untreated Gallstones

The consequences of delayed gallstone therapy can be severe and even fatal. Some of the potential issues are listed below:

Cholecystitis, or gallbladder inflammation, can be brought on by gallstones and result in stomach discomfort, fever, nausea, and vomiting.

Gallstones can also obstruct the bile duct, which can cause fever, stomach discomfort, and jaundice (a condition in which the skin and eyes turn yellow).

Gallstone blockage of the pancreatic duct can result in pancreatitis, an inflammation of the organ that can cause excruciating stomach pain, fever, and nausea.

Gallstones can clog the bile duct, which can result in cholangitis, a dangerous bacterial infection. Jaundice, chills, stomach discomfort, and fever are among the symptoms.

Gallbladder cancer: Although it's uncommon, gallstones might raise your chance of getting the disease.

In general, it's critical to seek medical assistance right away if you have any gallstone-related symptoms since rapid treatment can help avoid severe consequences.

CHAPTER FOUR: The Role of Diet in Gallstone Prevention and Management

Gallstones are compacted digestive fluid deposits that develop in the gallbladder, a tiny organ under the liver. If these stones obstruct the bile ducts or lodge in the gallbladder, they may result in excruciating pain, inflammation, and infection. While some individuals might not show any symptoms, others could need treatment, such as surgery to remove the stones.

Gallstone prevention and treatment are greatly influenced by diet. While some dietary components can assist to lower the risk of gallstone development, others can actually increase it. Following are some dietary suggestions for the treatment and prevention of gallstones:

Increase your intake of fiber: Fiber-rich foods including whole grains, fruits, and vegetables can help lower your chance of developing gallstones. The flow of waste through the digestive tract is aided by fiber, which also helps to control digestion.

Reduce your intake of meals with a lot of fat: Saturated and trans fats raise your chance of developing gallstones. Fried meals, fatty meats, and full-fat dairy products are a few examples of high-fat foods. Use lean protein alternatives instead, such fish, chicken, and beans.

Prevent fast weight loss: Gallstone development is increased by rapid weight loss brought on by excessive calorie restriction or fad diets. Instead, focus on slow, sustainable weight loss with a healthy diet and consistent exercise.

Keep hydrated: By preventing the bile secretions from getting too concentrated, drinking adequate water can help avoid the development of gallstones. Aim for 8 to 10 glasses of water a day, minimum.

Moderate alcohol consumption: Heavy drinking raises the risk of gallstone development. Alcohol consumption should be kept to a minimum, with women being advised to have one drink per day and males to have two.

Don't miss meals: Skipping meals or going without food for extended periods of time might raise the chance of gallstone development. For a smooth digestion, aim for regular meals and snacks throughout the day.

How diet affect Gallstones formation

There are several elements that can make one develop gallstones.
Diet is one of these elements..

Due to the fact that some meals can cause the production of these hardened deposits, diet has a substantial impact on the development of gallstones. Obesity, which is frequently associated with a diet heavy in fat and cholesterol, is one of the main risk factors for gallstones. Your body creates extra bile to aid in the breakdown of the fats you consume when you consume meals rich in cholesterol and fat. Gallstones may develop if there is an excessive buildup of cholesterol in the bile as a result of this.

Additionally, consuming a lot of sugar and refined carbohydrates can raise your risk of gallstones. These foods have the potential to quickly raise blood sugar levels, which may trigger an increase in the production of the hormone insulin. A rise in cholesterol synthesis brought on by high insulin levels may result in the development of gallstones.

In contrast, a diet low in fat and high in fiber can help lower your risk of gallstone development. Fruits, vegetables, and whole grains are examples of foods high in fiber that can help control your blood sugar levels and lower your risk of developing insulin resistance. Additionally, a low-fat diet can assist in lowering the level of cholesterol in your bile, which can aid in preventing the development of gallstones.

Additionally, some foods have been demonstrated to protect against gallstones. For instance, studies have demonstrated a link between gallstone risk reduction and moderate alcohol, caffeine, and coffee consumption. Coffee contains substances that can stimulate the gallbladder, thereby preventing bile buildup. Similar effects on the gallbladder have also been observed with caffeine, and moderate alcohol consumption lowers the risk of gallstones by enhancing liver function.

Finally, it can be said that diet significantly affects the development of gallstones. A diet that is high in fiber and low in fat can help lower your risk, while one that is low in fat and high in refined carbohydrates, sugar, and fat can increase your risk of developing these hardened deposits. In addition, some foods, including coffee, caffeine, and small amounts of alcohol, can help prevent gallstones. It is crucial to discuss dietary changes with your doctor if you are at risk of developing gallstones in order to lower that risk.

Food to eat to prevent Gallstone

Gallstones may be prevented in a big way by diet. Here we'll go through various meals that might help you avoid gallstones:

Fruits and veggies: Including fruits and vegetables in your diet can help you stay healthy. These meals have a low caloric intake and a high fiber content, both of which assist avoid gallstones. Antioxidants found in fruits and vegetables shield the body from the harm that free radicals may do. Moreover, they contain vitamin C, which aids in the bile's ability to breakdown cholesterol and prevents the development of gallstones.

Whole grains: Whole grains are rich in fiber, which can help avoid gallstones. Some examples of these grains are brown rice, quinoa, and whole wheat bread. Gallstone risk is decreased by fiber's ability to decrease the quantity of bile that is stored in the gallbladder. Magnesium, another component of whole grains, helps to prevent gallstones by lowering the amount of cholesterol the liver produces.

Consuming lean proteins like tofu, fish, and chicken can help avoid gallstones. Due to their minimal fat and calorie content, these meals aid in maintaining a healthy weight. Maintaining a healthy weight is crucial for preventing gallstones since obesity is a risk factor for the development of gallstones.

Low-fat dairy: Milk, yogurt, and cheese are examples of low-fat dairy foods that can help avoid gallstones. These meals provide calcium, which can stop cholesterol from accumulating in the bile ducts. Gallstone risk is decreased by calcium's role in the digestive system's breakdown of lipids.

Nuts and seeds: Consuming nuts and seeds might aid in gallstone prevention. These meals include a lot of fiber and good fats, which can help lower inflammation and stop cholesterol from accumulating in the bile ducts. The best options are walnuts, almonds, and sunflower seeds.

Coffee: Drinking coffee can aid in gallstone prevention. Caffeine, which is found in coffee, causes the gallbladder to constrict and discharge bile. Gallstone risk is decreased as a result of this strategy for preventing cholesterol accumulation in the gallbladder.

In summary, gallstones may be avoided by eating a diet high in fruits, vegetables, whole grains, lean meats, low-fat dairy, nuts, seeds, and coffee. Gallstones can be avoided by following a healthy diet, keeping a healthy weight, and drinking plenty of water.

Foods to avoid to prevent Gallstones

While certain meals can help prevent gallstones, others should be avoided in order to lower the chance of gallstone development. In order to avoid gallstones, you should steer clear of the following foods:

Foods that are rich in fat: Consuming foods that are high in fat, such as fried meals, fatty meats, and high-fat dairy products, might increase the chance of developing gallstones. Certain meals may increase the amount of cholesterol the liver produces, which may then accumulate in the bile ducts and result in the development of gallstones.

Foods that have been processed: Because processed foods like chips, crackers, and cookies are heavy in harmful fats and refined carbs, they raise the risk of gallstones. Moreover, these meals may contribute to obesity, which increases the risk of gallstones.

Sugary beverages: Sugary beverages, including soda, sports drinks, sweetened tea, and coffee, can raise the risk of gallstone development. These beverages include a lot of sugar and calories, which might cause obesity and increase the liver's synthesis of cholesterol.

Red meat: Red meat, especially beef and pig, might raise your risk of gallstones. Red meat has a lot of saturated fat, which can cause the liver to produce more cholesterol and raise the risk of gallstones.

White bread, white rice, and pasta produced from refined flour are examples of refined grains that might raise the risk of gallstones. These meals have little fiber and can elevate blood sugar levels, which can lead to obesity and enhance the liver's ability to produce cholesterol.

Alcohol: Consuming too much alcohol might make you more likely to have gallstones. Gallstones may form as a result of liver damage caused by alcohol and an increase in the liver's synthesis of cholesterol.

The chance of getting gallstones can be decreased by avoiding high-fat diets, processed foods, sugary beverages, red meat, refined cereals, and excessive alcohol use.

Gallstones can be avoided by eating a nutritious diet, keeping a healthy weight, and drinking plenty of water.

CHAPTER FIVE: The Gallstone Diet: Meal Planning and Preparation

TIPS FOR MEAL PLANNING

Planning your meals might be a significant part of controlling your gallstones if you have them. The following tips can help you make efficient meal plans:

Reduce your consumption of fat since eating foods high in fat can lead to gallbladder attacks. Steer clear of processed snacks, high-fat meats, and fried meals. Use lean meats, low-fat dairy products, and healthy fats like olive oil, almonds, and avocados as an alternative.

Eat modest, regular meals instead of big ones since doing so can help prevent gallbladder attacks and stress your digestive system. Try to replace it with modest, regular meals spread out throughout the day. This will ease pain and maintain a healthy digestive system.

Select high-fiber meals since they promote healthy digestion and can help ward against gallstones. Limit your consumption of processed carbs and sugar and place a greater emphasis on whole grains, fruits, and vegetables.

Keep hydrated: Water consumption is essential for avoiding gallstones. Drink at least eight glasses of water every day, and stay away from alcohol and sugary beverages.

Avoid trigger foods: Everyone has different triggers, but frequent triggers include dairy products, spicy meals, and coffee. See how your body responds to various foods, and steer clear of anything that looks to set off an attack.

Contact a trained dietitian: A registered dietitian may assist you in developing a customized meal plan that satisfies your dietary requirements and aids in the management of your gallstones. Also, they may offer advice on serving amounts, food preparation, and healthy cooking methods.

In conclusion, meal planning is crucial for gallstone management. You may establish a healthy, balanced diet that supports your digestive health and guards against gallbladder problems by heeding these recommendations and consulting a healthcare practitioner.

It's crucial to watch what you eat if you have gallstones in order to prevent gallbladder attacks. You can manage your diet by reading the nutrition labels, which is one useful tool. Here are some pointers on how to effectively read nutrition labels:

Start with the serving size: When reading a nutrition label, the serving size should be your first consideration. You can find out from this how much of the product constitutes a serving. This is significant because the information on the label is based on one serving, so you will need to adjust the numbers if you consume more than one serving.

Look at the calories: You should be aware of your calorie intake if you have gallstones because being overweight or obese increases your risk of developing gallstones. To aid in weight management, look for products with fewer calories.

Examine the fat content: The fat content is a crucial additional factor. Low-fat products are preferable because high-fat foods can cause gallbladder attacks. Pay attention to the amount of saturated and total fat.

Think about the cholesterol level: It's crucial to limit your intake of cholesterol because cholesterol is frequently a component of gallstones. Locate goods with lower cholesterol content.

Consider the amount of fiber in the food: Fiber is a crucial ingredient for digestive health and can help avoid gallstones. To encourage a healthy digestive system, choose goods with a greater fiber content.

Sugar and salt should also be taken into consideration as additional nutrients. Excessive salt consumption might raise your chance of getting gallstones whereas high sugar intake can cause weight gain. Seek for items that include less of these two nutrients.

Look at the list of ingredients: Lastly, check the product's ingredient list to discover what's within. To prevent gallbladder attacks, stay away from foods like processed meats, fried meals, and high-fat dairy items.

On that note,as a gallstone sufferer, checking nutrition labels may be a useful tool for regulating your diet. Be mindful of the serving sizes, calorie counts, fat, cholesterol, fiber, sugar, and salt content, as well as ingredient listings. You may simply and swiftly analyze items to choose those that are best for the health of your gallbladder with a little practice.

CHAPTER SIX:BREAKFAST RECIPE FOR GALLSTONES PATIENT

Gallstones may be excruciating and difficult, and controlling them frequently entails dietary adjustments. It's crucial for those who have gallstones to consume foods that are simple to digest and low in fat.

Gallstone-friendly breakfast options

Breakfast is a vital meal that is important to have every single day since it helps to rev up your metabolism for the day.

Here are some breakfast meal suggestions that are not only delicious and healthy, but also safe for folks who have gallstones.

Fruit-topped oatmeal: Prepare some basic porridge and garnish it with fresh berries, banana slices, or chopped apples. Because to its low fat content and high fiber content, oatmeal is simple to digest and can keep you satisfied until lunch.

Eggs scrambled with vegetables: Prepare some eggs scrambled with spinach, mushrooms, and onions that have been sautéed. This meal is a fantastic way to start the day because it is packed in protein and fiber.

Whole Wheat Toast with Almond Butter and Honey: For a wonderful and satisfying breakfast, spread some almond butter and honey over a slice of whole wheat bread. Because it contains a lot of protein and healthy fats, almond butter is a better choice than regular butter.

Greek yogurt smoothie: For a fast and simple morning smoothie, combine some Greek yogurt, frozen berries, and a little almond milk. Greek yogurt is a fantastic option for those who have gallstones since it is strong in protein and low in fat.

Breakfast burrito with black beans: For a wonderful and filling breakfast, wrap some scrambled eggs, black beans, and sliced tomatoes in a whole wheat tortilla. The whole wheat tortilla provides some nutritious carbs to the dish while the black beans are a fantastic source of protein and fiber.

Never forget to talk to your doctor or dietician before making any significant dietary adjustments. You may start your day off correctly while controlling your gallstones by integrating these breakfast recipe suggestions into your food plan.

Preparation instructions and cooking tips

In this line, we'll talk about the dietary guidelines for people with gallstones, including how their food should be prepared.

Limiting the consumption of specific types of lipids is the first step in treating gallstones via diet. Included in this are the trans fats, hydrogenated fats, and saturated fats that are frequently included in processed meals, fried dishes, and fatty meats. Patients should choose healthy fats instead, such those in avocados, nuts, seeds, and fatty fish.

Patients with gallstones should refrain from frying their meals when cooking. They should use healthier cooking techniques instead, such baking, grilling, or boiling. By using these techniques, the amount of additional fats and oils is kept to a minimum while the nutritional value of the meal is preserved.

Patients with gallstones can benefit greatly by steaming. With using less additional fats and oils, steaming aids in preserving the food's original flavor and texture. Furthermore, steaming is a fantastic way to prepare vegetables, which are a crucial component of any balanced diet.

Gallstone patients should be careful to stay away from high-fat dairy items such whole milk, cream, and cheese. Instead, they should choose dairy products that are low in fat or fat free, like skim milk, low-fat yogurt, and low-fat cheese.

Patients with gallstones should be careful to restrict their consumption of foods high in cholesterol in addition to monitoring their fat intake. This includes organ meats, fatty meats, and egg yolks. Lean meats like chicken, turkey, and fish, as well as egg whites, should be used as a substitute.

Patients with gallstones should refrain from flavoring their diet with heavy sauces or gravies that are high in fat. They should choose herbs and spices to flavor their dish instead. This helps them consume less additional fats and oils while also supplementing their diet with a range of phytonutrients that are good for their health.

Finally, those who have gallstones should be careful to minimize their consumption of certain fats and cholesterol, and they should choose healthier cooking techniques like baking, grilling, or steaming. Lean meats, low-fat dairy products, and vegetables should also be carefully chosen. In addition, people should season their food with herbs and spices rather than rich sauces or gravies. Patients can successfully control their gallstones and enhance their general health and well-being by adhering to these dietary suggestions.

Snacks Recipe for Gallstone diet

There are various recipes to take into account if you're seeking for a filling and nutritious snack choice that is also suitable for those with gallstones.

Roasted chickpeas are a fantastic meal for a snack for those with gallstones. Chickpeas are a wonderful source of fiber and protein in addition to a number of other minerals like iron, magnesium, and vitamin B6. Set your oven's temperature to 375°F before beginning to cook roasted chickpeas. A can of chickpeas should be rinsed and drained before being dried with paper towels. After that, distribute them on a baking sheet and sprinkle olive oil over them. Toss the chickpeas with your preferred ingredients, such as salt, pepper, and garlic powder, so they are equally coated. For 25 to 30 minutes, or until they are crispy and golden brown, roast the chickpeas in the oven. As a delightful and healthful snack, savor them.

Fruit salad is another another snack choice for those with gallstones. Fruits include a wealth of vitamins and minerals and can aid with digestion. Start by selecting a range of fruits that are low in fat and high in fiber, such berries, melons, and citrus fruits, to prepare a fruit salad. The fruits should be chopped into bite-sized pieces and combined in a basin. For additional taste, you may also use a drizzle of honey or a squeeze of lime juice. Fruit salad is a tasty and healthy snack that may be eaten at any time of the day.

Consider creating a hummus dip with veggies for a savory snack option. Chickpeas, which are a fantastic source of protein and fiber, are used to make hummus. To create the dip, combine a can of chickpeas with olive oil, garlic, lemon juice, and tahini in a food processor until it is smooth. Sliced veggies of your choosing, such as carrots, cucumbers, and bell peppers, should be served with the hummus dip. With this snack, you may increase the amount of veggies in your diet while simultaneously indulging in a delectable and nutritious dip.

That's to say, people with gallstones have a wide variety of delectable and nutritious snack choices. These dishes include healthy components like chickpeas, fruits, and veggies that can improve digestion and general wellbeing. There is a recipe to fit your taste preferences, whether you want salty or sweet treats. You may treat gallstones and enhance your general health by changing your diet and including nutritious snacks in it.

CHAPTER SEVEN: LUNCH RECIPE

There are various delectable and healthful choices to take into consideration when it comes to lunch meals for people with gallstones.

Quinoa and veggie salad is one lunchtime meal for those with gallstones. Quinoa has a high protein content, is high in fiber, and is low in fat and cholesterol. To create this salad, first prepare the quinoa as directed on the package. Mix the cooked quinoa with the veggies of your choosing, such as bell peppers, cherry tomatoes, and cucumbers. For additional flavor, mix in a few tablespoons of chopped herbs like parsley or cilantro. For a light and nutritious lunch alternative, drizzle the salad with olive oil and pour on a little lemon juice.

An additional lunch meal for those with gallstones is a stir-fry with chicken and vegetables. Vegetables are an excellent source of fiber and minerals, while chicken is a fantastic supply of protein. To begin preparing this recipe, brown the chicken breast on both sides on a nonstick pan. Then, add the veggies of your choosing, such as bell peppers, mushrooms, and broccoli, and sauté them until they are soft. For more taste, you may add your preferred seasonings, including soy sauce, ginger, and garlic. Turn the stir-fry into a substantial and healthy meal by serving it over a bed of brown rice.

Consider cooking lentil soup as a vegetarian dish. In addition to being a fantastic source of fiber and protein, lentils are also low in fat and cholesterol. Start by boiling the lentils in a saucepan with water, a bay leaf, and salt until they are soft. Then, add the veggies of your choosing, such carrots, celery, and onions, and sauté them until they are tender. For more taste, you may add your preferred seasonings, including cumin, coriander, and turmeric. For a warm and nutritious lunch, serve the soup with a slice of whole grain bread.

In conclusion, people with gallstones have a wide variety of enticing and healthful lunch alternatives. These dishes include healthy ingredients like quinoa, chicken, and lentils, which can improve digestion and general well-being. There is a dish to fit your tastes, whether you choose vegetarian or meat-based choices. You may treat gallstones and enhance your general health by changing your diet and including healthy lunch alternatives in it.

Dinner Recipe for gallstones patients

Grilled salmon and roasted veggies provide a delicious supper for people who have gallstones.
In addition to being a wonderful source of fiber and minerals, veggies are also a fantastic source of protein from salmon and omega-3 fatty

acids. Salmon fillets should first be seasoned with salt, pepper, and lemon juice before preparing this meal. The salmon should then be cooked all the way through on a hot grill. Roast your preferred veggies in the oven with a sprinkle of olive oil and your preferred spices while the salmon cooks, such as broccoli, asparagus, and sweet potatoes. Serve the cooked veggies and fish together for a satisfying and wholesome supper.

Turkey chili is an additional meal choice for those with gallstones. Beans are an excellent source of fiber, while turkey is a lean protein source. To begin making this chili, brown the ground turkey in a nonstick saucepan. Add your chosen veggies, such as tomatoes, peppers, onions, and black beans or kidney beans, after that. To enhance flavor, you may also add your preferred seasonings, including paprika, cumin, and chili powder. To enable the flavors to meld, let the chili simmer for at least 30 minutes. Serve the chili with a side of whole grain crackers or a slice of whole grain bread for a cozy and nutritious evening.

Make a tofu and veggie stir-fry as a vegetarian alternative. Vegetables are abundant in vitamins and fiber, and tofu is a fantastic source of protein. Start by squeezing the tofu firmly to squeeze out any extra water before preparing the meal. After that, cut the tofu into little cubes and brown both sides of it in a non-stick pan. Then, add your preferred veggies, including bell peppers, mushrooms, and broccoli, and sauté them until they are cooked. For more taste, season with your preferred ingredients, such as soy sauce, ginger, and garlic. For a hearty and wholesome meal, serve the stir-fry over a bed of brown rice or quinoa.

For those with gallstones, there are a variety of delectable and healthful meal alternatives. The healthy components used in these dishes, such salmon, turkey, tofu, and veggies, can aid with digestion and general well-being. There is a dish to fit your taste preferences, whether you choose meat-based or vegetarian choices. Gallstones may be controlled and your general health can be enhanced by dietary adjustments and the addition of healthy supper alternatives to your diet

Management Tips.
To cap this.
As a gallstones patient, it's important to manage your health wisely.
That's you have and must quit habits you think are unhealthy to you.
You also need to exercise frequently, avoid excessive alcohol and excessive smoking.

www.ingramcontent.com/pod-product-compliance
Lightning Source LLC
Chambersburg PA
CBHW072338270726
48659CB00022B/1894